PREGNANCY DIET COOKBOOK

I0479947

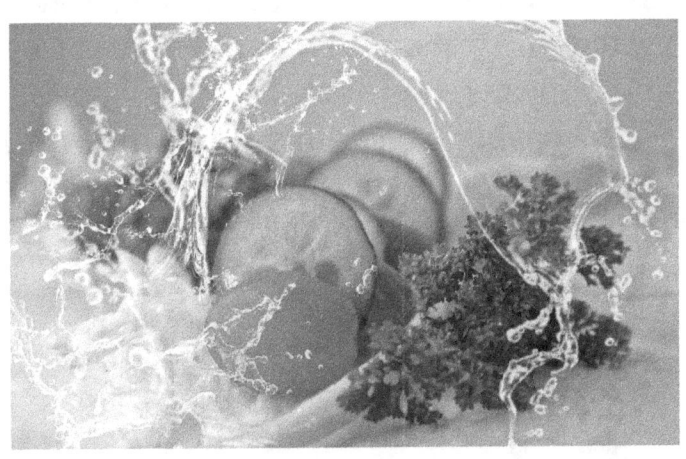

"Healthy Recipes to Help Nourish You and Your Baby During Pregnancy"

ANGELICA C.SILVERLAKE

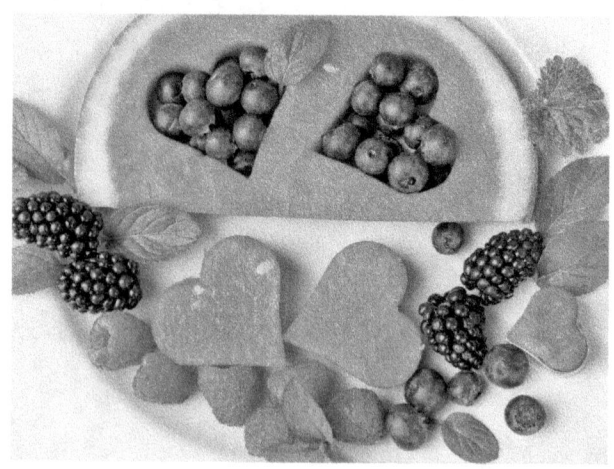

TABLE OF CONTENT

CONCLUSION   90

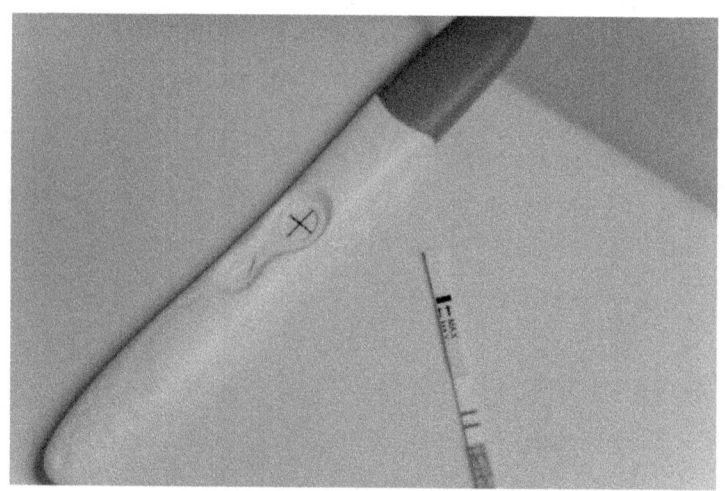

INTRODUCTION

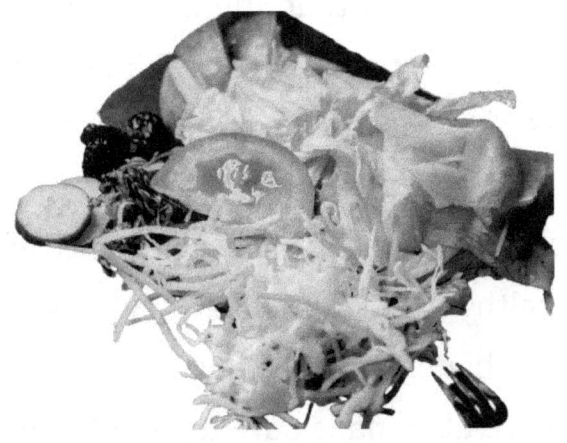

Claire was a newly pregnant woman and was excited to welcome her little bundle of joy into the world. She was determined to have a healthy pregnancy and wanted to make sure she was eating the right foods to give her baby the best start in life. She did her research and found this great pregnancy diet cookbook that she knew would help her during this special time in her life.

Claire was excited when she discovered that this pregnancy diet cookbook had recipes that were full of essential vitamins and minerals that she needed to support her and her baby's growth. She cooked up healthy meals every day, full of fresh fruits and vegetables, lean proteins, and whole grains. She also incorporated healthy snacks into her day so she could keep her cravings at bay.

Claire also made sure to get plenty of rest and exercise to keep her energy levels up and support her growing baby. She took long walks around the neighborhood, did yoga, and made sure to get enough sleep. She also made sure to stay hydrated throughout the day by drinking a lot of water.

This pregnancy diet cookbook was a lifesaver for Claire. She was able to stick to a healthy diet and keep her energy levels up. She felt great throughout her pregnancy and was able to give her baby the best start in life. Thanks to this amazing pregnancy diet cookbook, Claire was able to have a healthy and happy pregnancy.

A pregnancy diet cookbook is an invaluable resource for pregnant women looking to make healthy, nutritious meals for themselves and their growing baby. Pregnancy can be a time of tremendous physical, emotional, and dietary change, and having a cookbook full of nutrient-rich recipes can make the transition easier and more enjoyable.

This cookbook is designed to provide pregnant women with delicious and nutritious meals that will help to nourish both mother and baby. It contains recipes that are rich in essential vitamins, minerals, and other nutrients that are important for a healthy pregnancy. Recipes are also designed to provide enough calories to support the increased energy needs of the mother and her growing baby.

The recipes in this cookbook are divided into various categories, including breakfast, lunch, dinner, snacks, and desserts. Each category includes a variety of recipes that are easy to prepare and full of flavor. Many recipes are also suitable for vegetarians and those following other dietary restrictions.

For those who are new to cooking, the cookbook provides basic information on nutrition needs during pregnancy and tips on how to prepare and store food safely. It also includes a glossary of common ingredients and cooking techniques, as well as helpful advice and tips from experienced cooks.

This cookbook is an essential guide for any woman looking to make nutritious and delicious meals during her pregnancy. It provides a wide range of recipes to suit any taste and dietary needs, as well as helpful advice and information for those who are new to cooking. With this cookbook, pregnant women can confidently and easily create nutritious and tasty meals for themselves and their growing baby

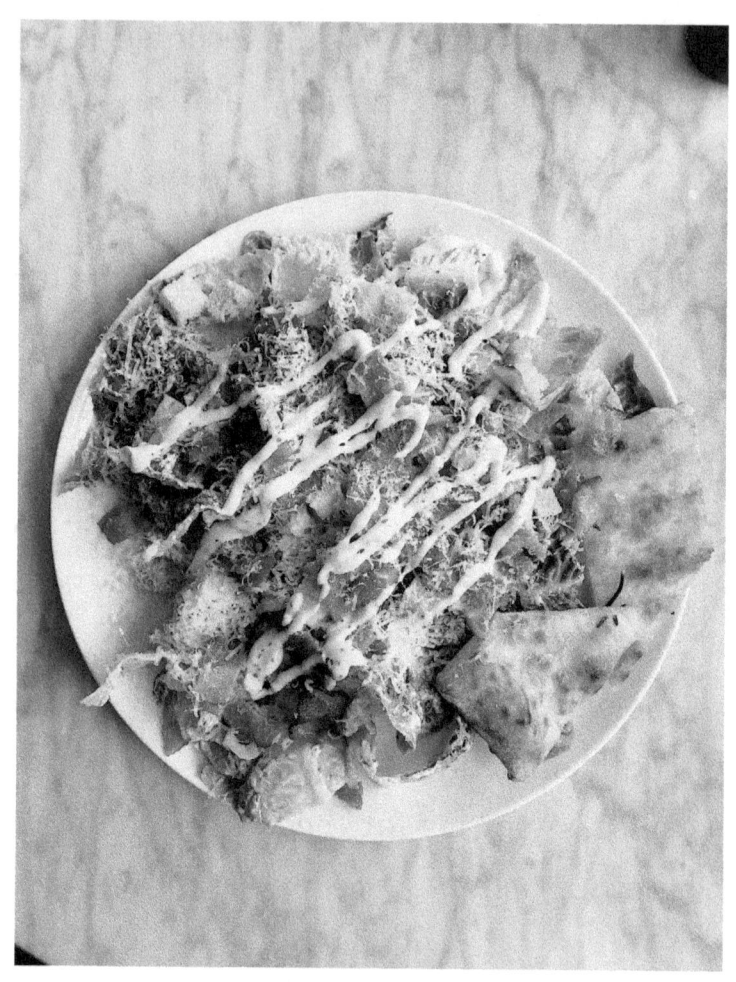

CHAPTER 1 :
Understanding Nutrition During Pregnancy

Pregnancy is an exciting time during which a woman's diet is especially important. Eating a nutritious and well-balanced diet during pregnancy is essential for the health of both mother and baby. Knowing what to eat and what to avoid can help ensure a healthy pregnancy.

Good nutrition during pregnancy is important for the proper growth and development of the baby. It is also important for the mother's health, as some pregnancy-related conditions such as anemia and gestational diabetes can be linked to poor nutrition.

A pregnant woman should aim to eat a wide variety of healthy foods from all the food groups. Eating a variety of foods ensures that the mother and baby get all the vitamins, minerals, and other nutrients they need.

In general, pregnant women should aim to consume an extra 300 calories per day. This should come from nutrient-dense foods like fruits, vegetables, whole grains, lean proteins, and healthy fats.

In addition to a balanced diet, it is important to take a prenatal vitamin to ensure that the mother and baby are getting all the necessary nutrients. Iron, folic acid, and calcium are especially important during pregnancy

It is important to avoid certain foods during pregnancy, as some can increase the risk of food-borne illness. These include raw and undercooked meats, unpasteurized dairy products, raw eggs, and certain types of seafood. Alcohol and caffeine should also be avoided, as they can have negative effects on the baby's development.

Overall, good nutrition during pregnancy is essential for the health of both mother and baby. Eating a variety of nutrient-dense foods, taking a prenatal vitamin, and avoiding certain foods can help ensure a healthy pregnancy. With the right nutrition and care, the mother and baby can have a healthy and happy pregnancy.

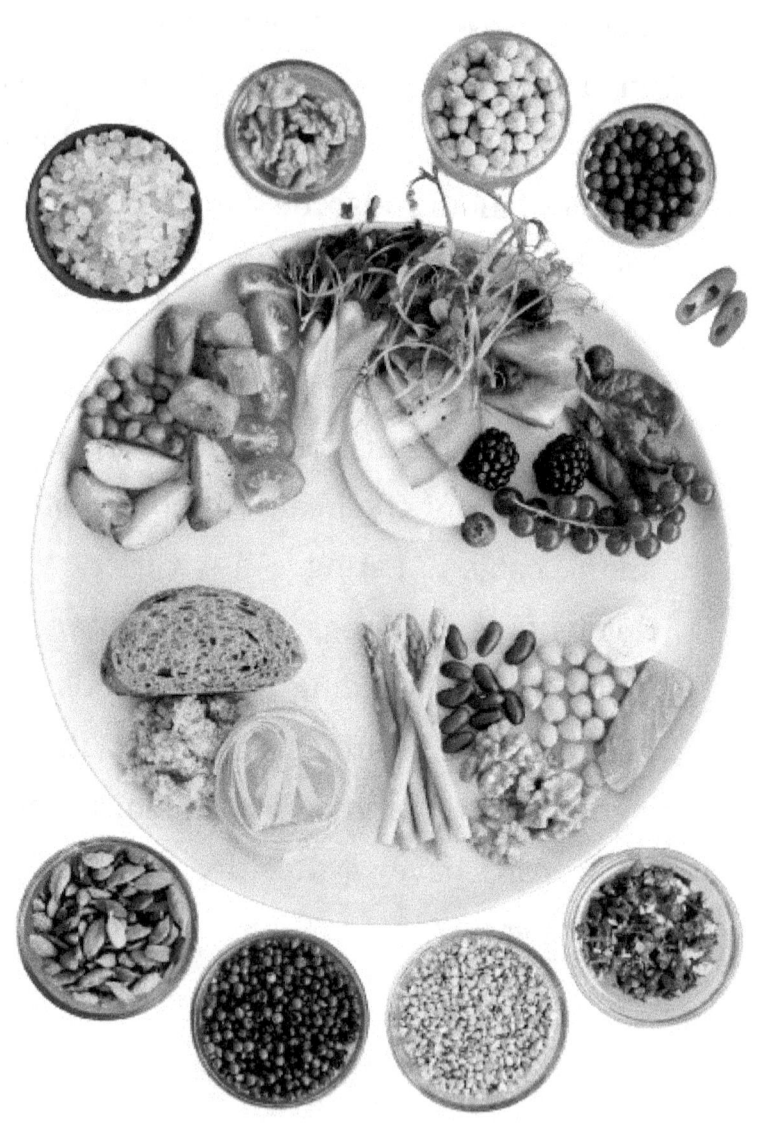

CHAPTER 2: Eating For Two-Nutritional Needs During Pregnancy

When you're pregnant, you need to make sure that you are eating healthy and getting all the nutrients both you and your baby need. Eating for two means that you need to increase your caloric intake, focus on eating nutrient-dense foods, and avoid certain foods.

The extra calories you need during pregnancy will depend on your weight before you become pregnant. Generally, women who had a BMI between 19-25 are recommended to consume an extra 340 calories per day during the second trimester and 452 calories per day during the third trimester. Women who had a BMI of 26 or greater before becoming pregnant are recommended to consume an extra 452 calories per day during the second trimester and 548 calories per day during the third trimester.

It's important to focus on eating nutrient-dense foods that are rich in vitamins and minerals like fruits, vegetables, whole grains, healthy fats, and lean proteins. You should also drink plenty of fluids and aim to get at least seven hours of sleep each night.

Here are some specific nutrient needs you should focus on during your pregnancy:

Folate: Folate is a B vitamin that helps protect against birth defects. It is important to get enough folate, especially during the first trimester of pregnancy. Good sources of folate include dark leafy greens, beans, and fortified grains.

Calcium: Calcium helps build strong bones and teeth for both you and your baby. Good sources of calcium include dairy products, fortified juices, and dark leafy greens.

Iron: Iron helps your body make the extra red blood cells it needs to support your growing baby. You can get iron from lean meats, fortified cereals, beans, and dark leafy greens.

Vitamin D: Vitamin D helps your body absorb calcium and is important for your baby's bone development. You can get vitamin D from fortified foods, such as milk and orange juice, and from exposing your skin to the sun.

Protein: Protein helps build the muscles and organs of your baby and can also help you maintain a healthy weight during pregnancy. Good sources of protein include lean meats, beans, nuts, and eggs.

Omega-3 fatty acids: Omega-3 fatty acids are essential fatty acids that are important for the development of your baby's brain and nervous system. You can get omega-3s from fatty fish like salmon, tuna, and mackerel, as well as from flaxseed and nuts. It's important to talk to your doctor about taking a supplement if you don't get enough omega-3s in your diet.

It's important to make sure you're getting enough of these essential nutrients during pregnancy. Eating a balanced diet and talking to your doctor about any supplements you may need can help ensure you and your baby stay healthy.

There are also certain foods that you should avoid during pregnancy, including raw meats, unpasteurized dairy products, and certain fish that may contain high levels of mercury. It's also important to limit your caffeine intake and avoid alcohol entirely.

Overall, it's important to eat a balanced, nutrient-dense diet during pregnancy to ensure that you and your baby are getting the nutrition you both need.

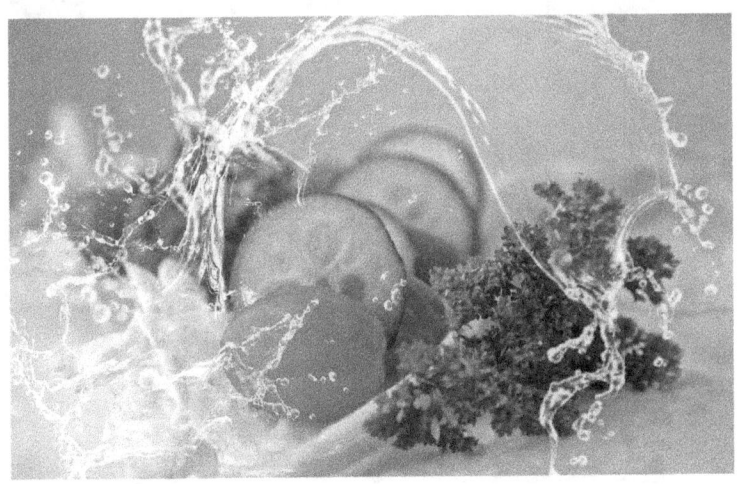

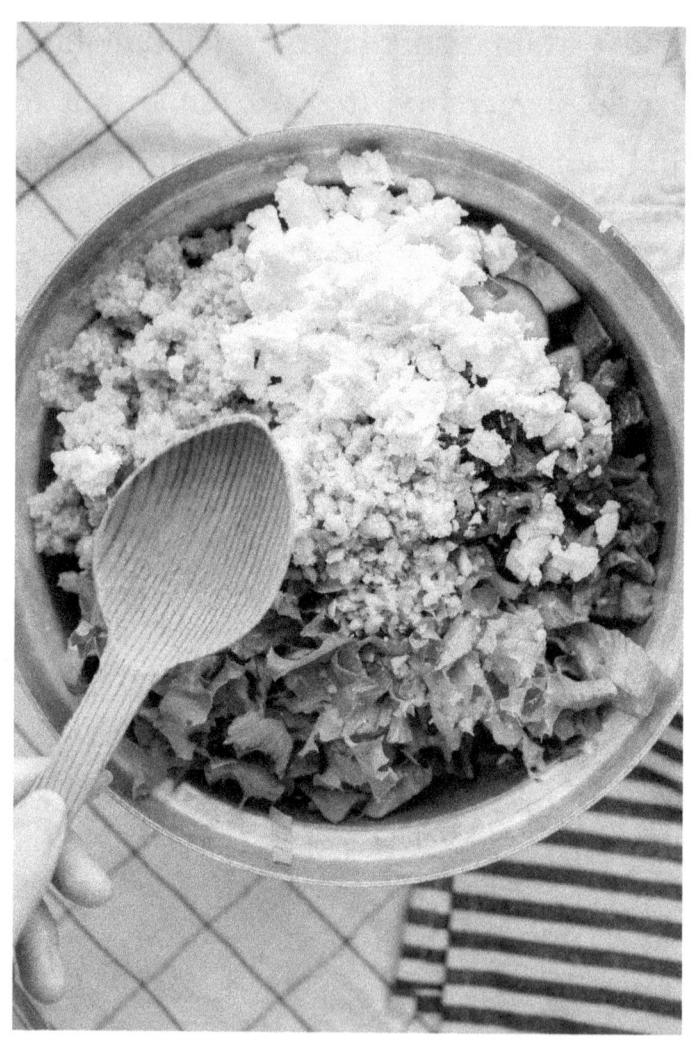

CHAPTER 3: Morning Sickness And Healthy Eating

Morning sickness is a common pregnancy symptom experienced by almost 75% of pregnant women. It is characterized by feelings of nausea, vomiting, and sometimes even dizziness. Although morning sickness usually subsides after the first trimester, it can be uncomfortable and even debilitating for some women during the first few months. Eating a healthy diet is one of the most important things you can do to manage morning sickness.

The key to managing morning sickness is to limit the intake of foods that can cause it. Foods that are high in fat, acidic, spicy, or heavily seasoned can all contribute to an increased risk of nausea and vomiting during pregnancy. Eating smaller meals more frequently throughout the day can also help, as it can keep your blood sugar levels steady and prevent nausea.

Having a variety of nutritious foods at your disposal can also help to reduce morning sickness. Eating a balanced diet of complex carbohydrates, lean proteins, and healthy fats is important, as it will provide your body with all the necessary nutrients it needs to stay healthy during pregnancy. Complex carbohydrates such as whole grains and legumes can help provide a steady release of energy throughout the day, while lean proteins like fish and poultry can help provide a feeling of fullness that can last longer and prevent nausea. Eating plenty of fruits and vegetables can also provide needed vitamins and minerals to help your baby grow.

To stay hydrated during pregnancy is very important . Dehydration can worsen the symptoms of morning sickness, so drinking plenty of fluids throughout the day is essential. Water is always the best choice, but other fluids like coconut water and low-sugar juices can also be helpful. Avoiding caffeine and limiting your intake of sugary drinks can also help reduce symptoms of morning sickness.

Finally, getting plenty of rest is important for managing morning sickness. Try to get as much rest as possible, as sleep can help to reduce the feelings of nausea. Taking time to relax and practice deep breathing can also help to reduce stress and ease nausea.

By following these simple guidelines, you can help to manage the symptoms of morning sickness and ensure that you are getting the nutrition your body needs during pregnancy. Eating a healthy diet, staying hydrated, and getting plenty of rest can all help to reduce the symptoms of morning sickness and ensure that you and your baby remain healthy throughout your pregnancy.

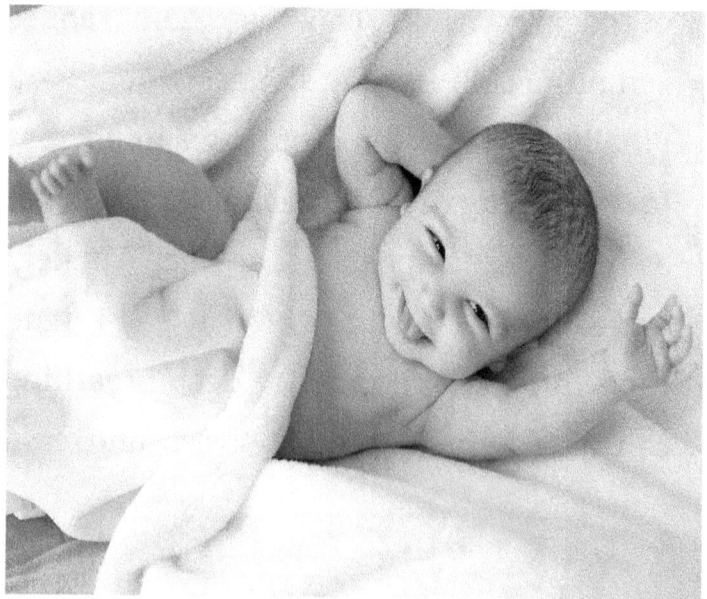

CHAPTER 4:
Creating A Balanced Diet During Pregnancy

Pregnancy is an exciting time, but it also requires extra nutrition and care. Eating a balanced diet during pregnancy is essential for your baby's development and your own health. Here are some tips for creating a healthy, balanced diet during pregnancy.

1. **Eat a variety of foods:** To get all the nutrients you and your baby need, it's important to eat a variety of foods from all the food groups. These include fruits, vegetables, whole grains, lean proteins, low-fat dairy, and healthy fats.

2. **Include plenty of fiber:** Fiber is important for maintaining regularity and

preventing constipation, which is common during pregnancy. Aim for 25-30 grams of fiber per day from sources like fruits, vegetables, whole grains, and legumes.

3. **Include foods rich in iron and folic acid:** Iron and folic acid are important nutrients for pregnant women. Iron helps form hemoglobin, which carries oxygen to your baby's cells. Folic acid helps reduce the risk of neural tube defects. Good sources of iron include lean red meat, dark leafy greens, and beans. Folic acid is found in leafy greens, citrus fruits, and fortified cereals.

4. **Limit processed and sugary foods :** Processed foods, such as canned soups, frozen dinners, and chips, are usually high in sodium and unhealthy fats. Limit these foods and instead focus on nutrient-dense whole foods. Additionally, too much sugar

can lead to unhealthy weight gain and other complications. Choose healthy snacks like fruits, nuts, and yogurt instead.

5. **Drink plenty of fluids**: Staying hydrated is essential during pregnancy. Aim for eight 8-ounce glasses of water each day. You can also get fluids from other beverages like milk, juice, and herbal teas.

Eating a balanced diet during pregnancy is essential for your health and your baby's development. Focus on eating a variety of nutrient-dense foods and limiting processed and sugary foods. If you're having trouble planning your meals or have nutrition-related questions, talk to your healthcare provider for personalized advice.

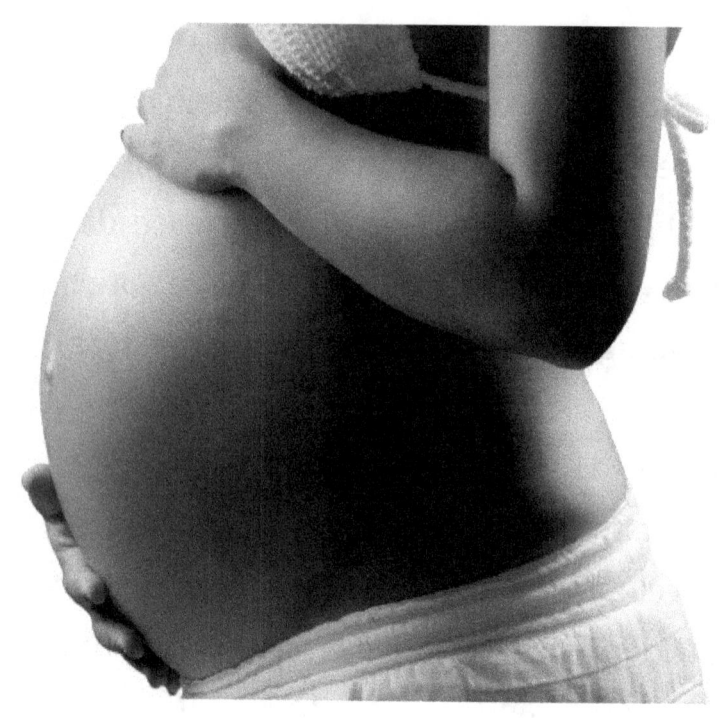

CHAPTER 5

Eating For Two On A Budget

Eating for two on a budget can be a difficult task for an expecting mother. With the cost of groceries and other items going up, many mothers-to-be struggle to maintain a nutritious diet while also staying within their budget. Here are some tips for expecting mothers to enjoy a healthy diet on a budget:

1. Plan your meals in advance: Planning meals in advance helps you to avoid impulse buys and stick to your grocery list. Make a list of meals you plan to make for the week, and shop for the ingredients you need ahead of time. This can help you save money by avoiding over-buying and wasting food.

2. Buy in bulk: Buying in bulk can be a great way to save money on food. Look for items like grains, beans, nuts, and canned goods that you can buy in bulk and store for long periods of time. This can help you save money and also ensure that you have healthy staples on hand.

3. Buy frozen produce: Frozen produce can be a good option for expecting mothers on a budget. Frozen fruits and vegetables are often cheaper than fresh and can last longer, so you don't have to worry about them going bad.

4. Take advantage of coupons and discounts: Many grocery stores offer discounts and coupons for expecting mothers. Check your local grocery store for special offers and take advantage of them whenever possible.

5. Shop seasonally: Shopping for fruits and vegetables in season can be a great way to save money. Not only are in-season produce items typically cheaper, but they're also more likely to be fresher and of higher quality.

6. Buy generic: Generic products are often cheaper than name-brand items, and they can be just as nutritious. Look for generic versions of items like grains, beans, and other pantry staples to save money.

7. Look for sales: Many grocery stores have weekly or monthly sales on items like fruits and vegetables. Take advantage of these sales to save money on produce and other healthy items.

Eating for two on a budget doesn't have to be difficult. With a little planning and creativity, expecting mothers can enjoy a nutritious diet while staying within their budget.

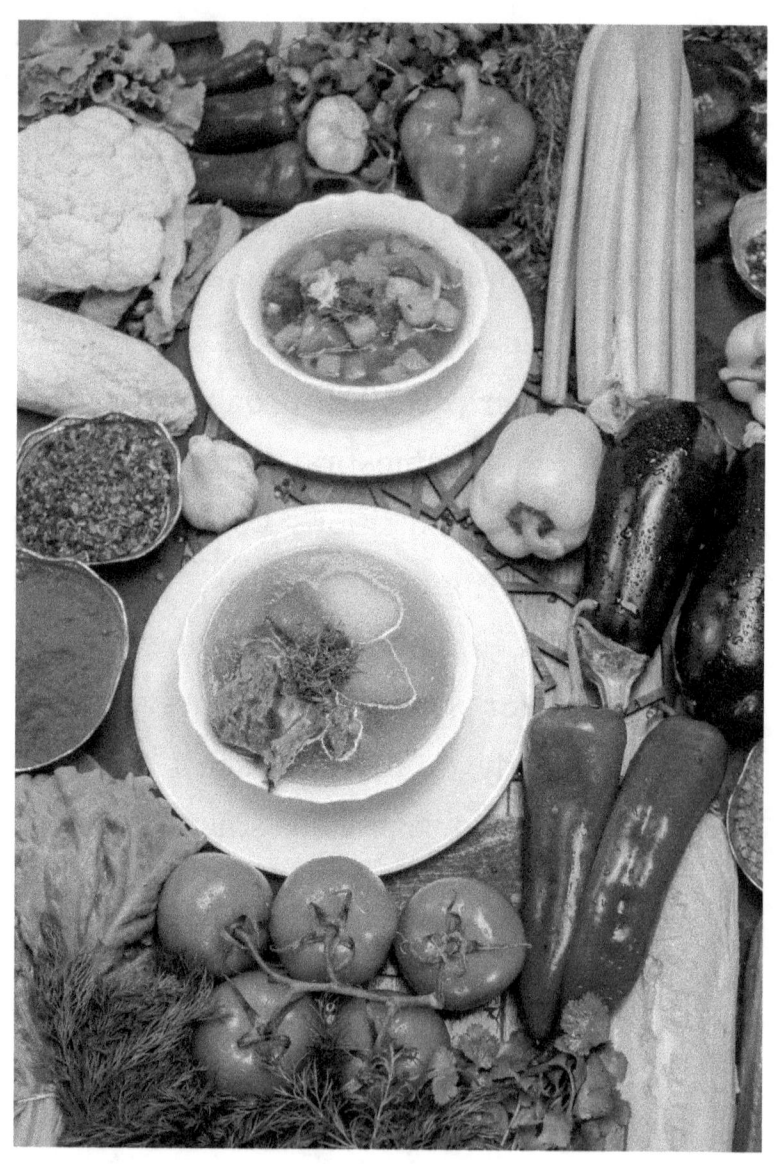

CHAPTER 6:Eating Well During Pregnancy

Eating well during pregnancy is an important part of ensuring the health and wellbeing of both mother and baby. What you eat can affect your baby's growth and development, and your own health. Pregnant women need to eat a balanced and varied diet that includes a wide range of foods from the five main food groups: fruits and vegetables, grains, dairy, protein and healthy fats.

Here are some tips for eating well during pregnancy:

1. **Eat a variety of foods.** Eating a wide variety of foods from all five food groups will ensure you get the essential nutrients you and your baby need. Choose foods that are high in vitamins, minerals and fiber,

such as fruits and vegetables, whole grains, lean proteins, low-fat dairy products and healthy fats.

2. **Increase your calorie intake.** You need extra calories during pregnancy to ensure your baby has all the nutrients they need to grow and develop. Aim for an extra 300-500 calories a day.

3. **Eat small, frequent meals.** Eating small, frequent meals throughout the day can help keep your energy levels and blood sugar levels stable, and prevent nausea.

4. **Avoid certain foods and drinks.** Some foods and drinks are unsafe to consume during pregnancy and should be avoided, such as raw or undercooked meats, unpasteurised dairy products, and certain types of fish. Additionally, you should avoid alcohol and caffeine.

5. **Stay hydrated**. Drinking plenty of water is important for your own health, as well

as your baby's. Aim to drink at least 8 glasses of water a day.

Eating a nutritious, balanced diet during pregnancy is important for both you and your baby's health. By following the tips outlined above, you can ensure you are getting all the essential nutrients you need to stay healthy and help your baby grow and develop.

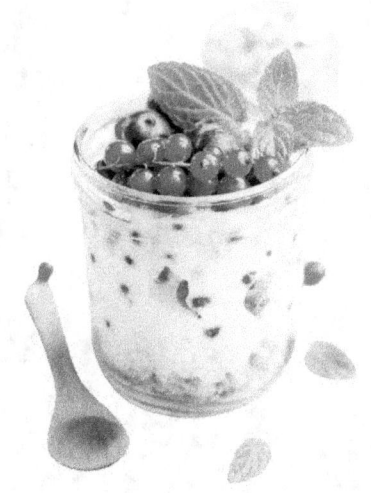

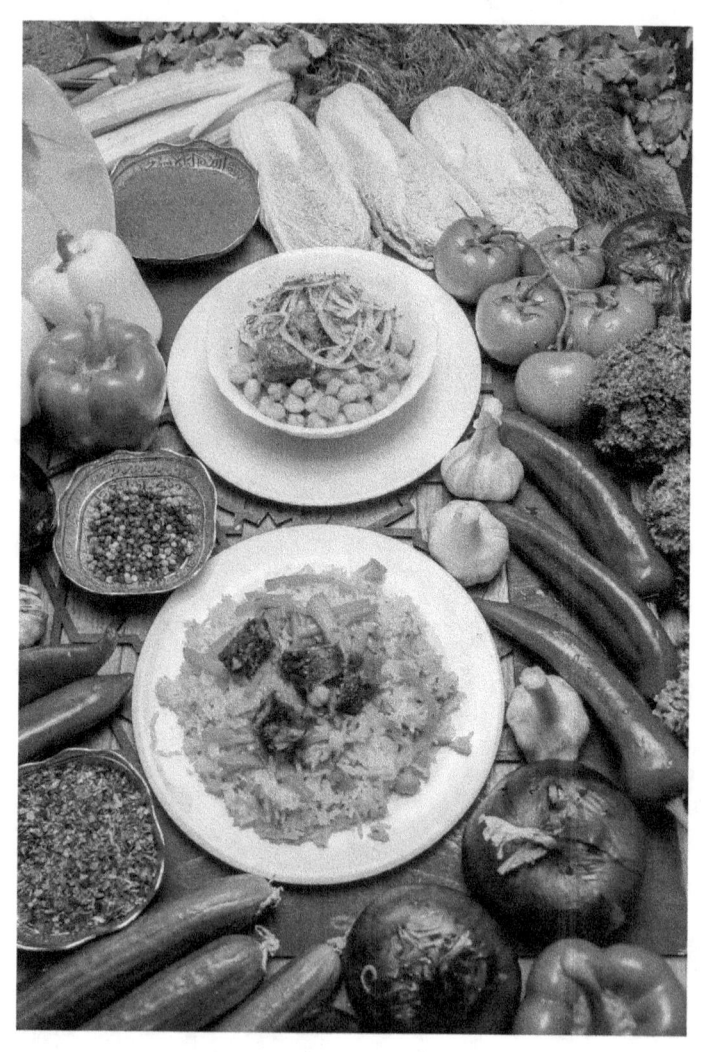

CHAPTER 7:Healthy Meal Plan For Pregnant Woman

A healthy meal plan for pregnant women is essential to ensure that both mother and baby are getting the nutrients they need. While pregnant women require additional calories and nutrients to support the growth of their baby, it is important to make sure that the food choices are healthy and provide the essential nutrients for a healthy pregnancy.

What To Eat

Pregnant women should focus on eating a variety of nutritious foods from all of the food groups. The following is a list of healthy foods that should be included in a pregnant woman's diet:

• **Fruits and vegetables:** Aim for at least 5-7 servings of fruits and vegetables daily. These should be varied and include dark leafy greens, citrus fruits, red and yellow vegetables.

• **Whole grains:** Choose whole grain breads, cereals, and pastas to ensure adequate fiber intake.

• **Protein:** Choose lean proteins such as beans, fish, poultry, and eggs.

• **Dairy:** Aim for 3-4 servings of low-fat dairy daily.

• **Healthy fats:** Choose healthy fats such as nuts, seeds, avocados, and olive oil.

Tips for Eating Healthy During Pregnancy

• Eat 3 meals and 2-3 snacks

- Make each meal and snack balanced with a combination of carbohydrates, proteins, and fats
- Eat a variety of colors and textures
- Include a source of protein at each meal
- Eat foods rich in iron, folate, and calcium
- Stay hydrated with water
- Avoid processed and sugary foods

What Not to Eat

It is important for pregnant women to avoid certain foods and beverages that may pose a risk to the baby. The following is a list of foods that should be avoided during pregnancy:
- Unpasteurized soft cheeses
- Raw or undercooked fish or eggs
- Raw sprouts
- Unwashed fruits and vegetables
- Alcohol
- Some deli meats and hot dogs

• Caffeine

• Certain types of fish that are high in mercury

Eating a healthy and balanced diet during pregnancy is essential for the health of both the mother and baby. Pregnant women should aim to eat a variety of foods from all the food groups and limit processed and sugary foods. It is also important to avoid certain foods and beverages that could put the baby at risk. Eating healthy and following a nutritious meal plan can help ensure a healthy and successful pregnancy.

7 Days Pregnancy Meal Plan

Day 1

Breakfast: Oatmeal made with milk and topped with almonds and berries.

Lunch: Quinoa and vegetable stir-fry.

Snack: Greek yogurt with chia seeds and fresh fruit.

Dinner: Baked salmon with asparagus and brown rice.

Day 2

Breakfast: Scrambled eggs with spinach and roasted tomatoes.

Lunch: Kale salad with grilled chicken and roasted sweet potatoes.

Snack: Apple slices with peanut butter.

Dinner: Baked cod with roasted broccoli and quinoa.

Day 3

Breakfast: Whole wheat toast with avocado and poached eggs.

Lunch: Lentil soup with a side of grilled vegetables.

Snack: Celery sticks with hummus.

Dinner: Grilled chicken with roasted Brussels sprouts and a sweet potato.

Day 4

Breakfast: Vegetable frittata with a side of whole wheat toast.

Lunch: Turkey wrap with spinach and tomatoes.

Snack: Banana smoothie.

Dinner: Baked salmon with roasted asparagus and wild rice.

Day 5

Breakfast: Oatmeal pancakes topped with blueberries.

Lunch: Quinoa and black bean salad.

Snack: Greek yogurt and fresh fruit.

Dinner: Grilled chicken with roasted sweet potatoes and broccoli.

Day 6

Breakfast: Toast with peanut butter and banana.

Lunch: Grilled chicken wrap with lettuce and tomatoes.

Snack: Apple slices with almond butter.

Dinner: Baked cod with roasted vegetables and quinoa.

Day 7

Breakfast: Scrambled eggs with spinach and roasted tomatoes.

Lunch: Kale and quinoa salad.

Snack: Carrot sticks with hummus.

Dinner: Baked tofu with roasted Brussels sprouts and brown rice.

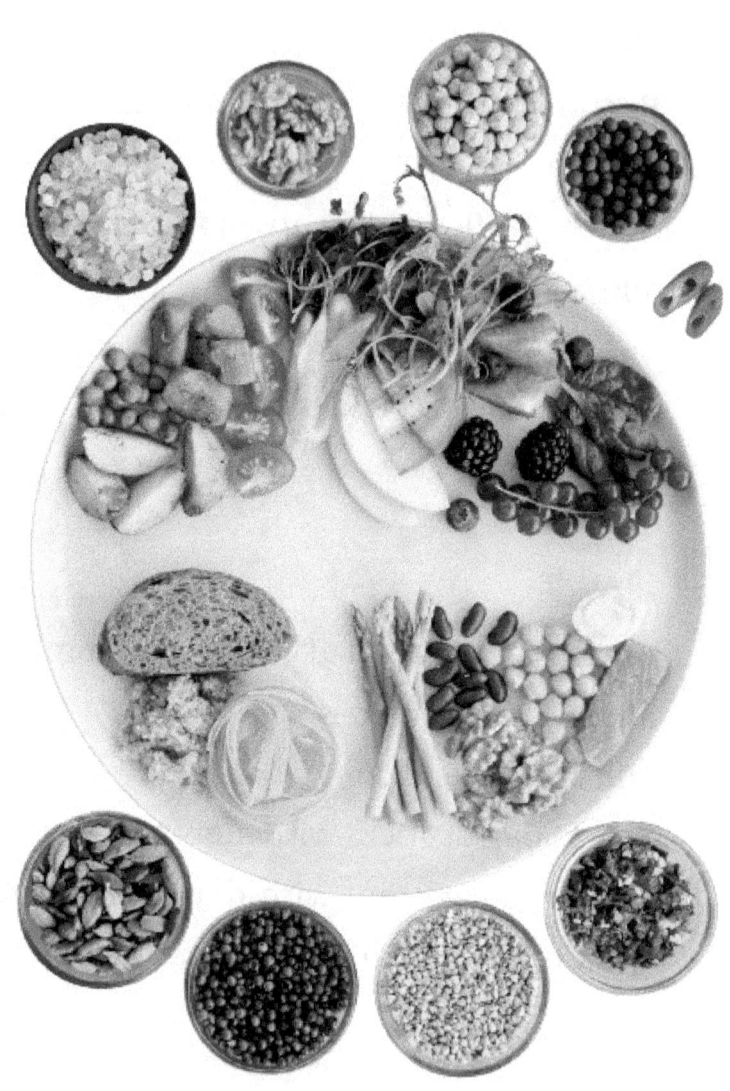

46

CHAPTER 8

Healthy Pregnancy Recipes

Breakfast

1. Spinach and Feta Frittata:

Ingredients:

2 tablespoons olive oil

2 cloves garlic (minced),

1 cup baby spinach leaves

4 large eggs

1/4 cup crumbled feta cheese

Salt and black pepper to taste

Instructions:

Preheat the oven to 375 degrees F. Heat olive oil over medium heat in a 10-inch oven-safe skillet. Add garlic and cook for 1 minute. Add spinach and cook for 1 minute. In a medium bowl, whisk together eggs, feta cheese, salt, and pepper. Pour egg mixture over spinach and stir until evenly combined. Cook for 5 minutes, stirring occasionally. Place the skillet in a preheated oven and bake for 10 minutes, or until eggs are cooked through. Serve warm.

Prep Time: 15 minutes

2. Avocado Toast:

Ingredients:

2 slices of whole grain bread

1 ripe avocado

Juice of 1/2 lemon

2 teaspoons olive oil

Salt and black pepper to taste

Instructions:

Toast bread until golden. Meanwhile, mash avocado in a bowl and season with

lemon juice, olive oil, salt, and pepper.
Spread mashed avocado over toast and
enjoy.

Prep Time: 5 minutes

3. Yog Parfait:

Ingredients:
1 cup plain Greek yogurt
1/2 cup granola
1/4 cup fresh berries
Instructions:
In a bowl, layer yogurt, granola, and
berries. Enjoy!
Prep Time: 5 minutes

4. Overnight Oats:

Ingredients:

1/2 cup rolled oats

1/2 cup milk of choice

1/2 teaspoon ground cinnamon

1/4 cup plain Greek yogurt

1 tablespoon honey

1/4 cup fresh or frozen fruit

Instructions:

In a bowl, combine oats, milk, and cinnamon. Cover and refrigerate overnight. In the morning, stir in yogurt and honey. Top with fruit and enjoy.

Prep Time: 10 minutes (plus overnight)

5. Berry Smoothie:

Ingredients:

1 cup frozen mixed berries, 1/2 cup plain Greek yogurt, 1/2 cup milk of choice, 1 tablespoon honey

Instructions: Place all ingredients in a blender and blend until smooth. Serve immediately.

Prep Time: 5 minutes

6. Egg and Avocado Sandwich:

Ingredients:

2 slices of whole grain bread

1 ripe avocado

1 large hard boiled egg (sliced)

Salt and black pepper to taste

Instructions:

Toast bread until golden. Meanwhile, mash avocado in a bowl and season with salt and pepper. Spread mashed avocado over toast and top with sliced egg. Enjoy.

Prep Time: 5 minutes

7. Peanut Butter and Banana Toast:

Ingredients:

2 slices of whole grain bread

2 tablespoons peanut butter

1 ripe banana (sliced)

Instructions: Toast bread until golden. Spread peanut butter over toast and top with banana slices. Enjoy.

Prep Time: 5 minutes

8. Sweet Potato Toast:

Ingredients:

2 slices of whole grain bread

1/2 cup mashed cooked sweet potato

Instructions: Toast bread until golden. Spread mashed sweet potato over toast. Enjoy.

Prep Time: 5 minutes

9. Apple and Almond Butter Toast:

Ingredients:

2 slices of whole grain bread

2 tablespoons almond butter, 1/2 apple (sliced)

Instructions: Toast bread until golden. Spread almond butter over toast and top with sliced apple. Enjoy.

Prep Time: 5 minutes

10. Egg Muffins:

Ingredients:

4 large eggs

1/4 cup chopped bell pepper

1/4 cup chopped onion

1/4 cup shredded cheese

Salt and black pepper

Instructions:

Preheat the oven to 375 degrees F. Grease a muffin tin with cooking spray. In a bowl, whisk together eggs, bell pepper, onion, cheese, salt, and pepper. Pour egg mixture into muffin tin, filling each cup about halfway. Bake for 15 minutes, or until eggs are cooked through. Serve warm.

Prep Time: 15 minutes

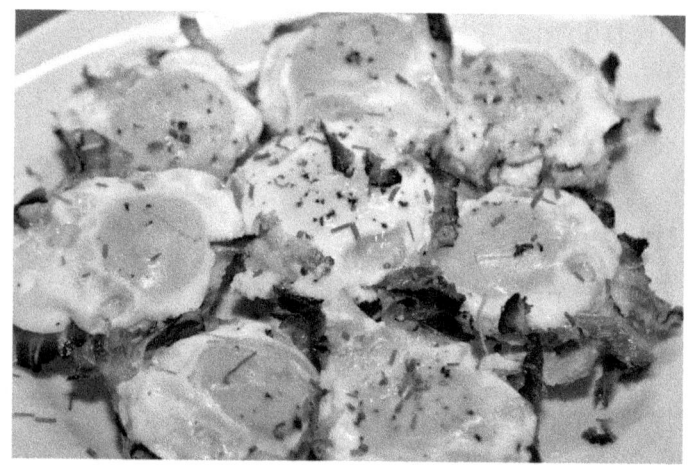

CHAPTER 9:

Healthy Pregnancy Recipe

Lunch

1.Grilled Chicken and Veggie Salad:

Ingredients:

1/2 cup cooked chicken breast,

1/2 cup cooked quinoa

1/2 cup cooked vegetables of your choice
(e.g., carrots, peppers, broccoli)

1/4 cup feta cheese

1/4 cup olive oil

1 tablespoon red wine vinegar

salt and pepper to taste.

Instructions:

Preheat the oven to 350 degrees Fahrenheit. Cook the chicken breast in a greased skillet over medium heat until it's cooked through. Cook the quinoa and vegetables in boiling water for 10 minutes. Place the cooked chicken, quinoa and vegetables in a large bowl and mix with the feta cheese, olive oil, red wine vinegar, salt and pepper. Place the salad in a greased baking dish and bake for 15 minutes. Serve warm or cold.

Prep time: 25 minutes

2. Egg Salad Sandwich:

Ingredients:

2 hard boiled eggs,

2 tablespoons mayonnaise

1 tablespoon whole-grain mustard,

1/4 teaspoon garlic powder

2 slices whole-wheat bread

lettuce, tomato and onion slices.

Instructions:

Peel and mash the eggs in a medium-sized bowl. Stir in the mayonnaise mustard and garlic powder. Spread the mixture on one slice of bread. Top with lettuce, tomato and onion slices. Top with the second slice of bread and serve.

Prep time: 15 minutes

3. Chicken Avocado Wrap:

Ingredients:

2 ounces cooked chicken breast,

1/4 avocado

1/4 cup shredded lettuce

1/4 cup diced tomatoes

1/4 cup diced cucumbers

2 tablespoons hummus, 1 whole wheat wrap.

Instructions:

Place the cooked chicken breast, avocado, lettuce, tomatoes, and cucumbers in the center of the wrap. Spread the hummus over the top. Roll up the wrap and cut in half. Serve

Prep time: 10 minutes

4. Spinach and Feta Frittata:

Ingredients:

2 tablespoons olive oil

1 small onion, diced

2 cloves garlic, minced

1/2 teaspoon dried oregano

1/2 teaspoon dried basil

1/4 teaspoon red pepper flakes

1/2 teaspoon salt

1/2 teaspoon black pepper

2 cups baby spinach

8 large eggs

1/2 cup crumbled feta cheese.

Instructions:

Preheat the oven to 350 degrees Fahrenheit. Heat the olive oil in a large skillet over medium heat. Add the onion, garlic, oregano, basil, red pepper flakes, salt and pepper. Sauté until the onion is softened. Add the spinach and cook until wilted. In a large bowl, whisk together the eggs and feta cheese. Pour the egg mixture into the skillet and gently stir to combine. Transfer the skillet to the oven and bake for 20 minutes. Let cool before slicing and serving.

Prep time: 25 minutes

5. Tuna Salad Lettuce Wraps:

Ingredients:

1 can tuna, drained

2 tablespoons mayonnaise

1 tablespoon diced onion

1/2 teaspoon dijon mustard

1/4 teaspoon garlic powder

4 large lettuce leaves

1/4 cup diced tomatoes.

Instructions:

In a medium bowl, mix together the tuna, mayonnaise, onion, dijon mustard, and garlic powder. Divide the mixture among the lettuce leaves. Top with the diced tomatoes. Roll up the lettuce leaves and enjoy.

Prep time: 10 minutes

6. Quinoa and Black Bean Burrito Bowl:

Ingredients:

1/2 cup cooked quinoa,

1/4 cup cooked black beans,

1/4 cup salsa,

1/4 cup diced avocado,

1/4 cup corn,

1 tablespoon chopped cilantro,

1/2 teaspoon chili powder,

1/4 teaspoon cumin,

2 tablespoons of low-fat Greek yogurt.

Instructions:

Place the cooked quinoa in a bowl. Top with the cooked black beans, salsa, avocado, corn, cilantro, chili powder, and cumin. Stir to combine. Top with the Greek yogurt. Serve.

Prep time: 10 minutes

7. Turkey and Cheese Sandwich:

Ingredients :

2 slices whole-wheat bread,

2 ounces deli turkey,

2 slices cheese of your choice,

1 tablespoon mayonnaise,

1 tablespoon mustard, lettuce and tomato slices.

Instructions:

Spread the mayonnaise and mustard on one slice of bread. Top with the turkey, cheese, lettuce and tomato. Top with the second slice of bread and serve.

Prep time: 5 minutes

8. Greek Yogurt Parfait:

Ingredients:

1/2 cup plain Greek yogurt

1/4 cup granola

1/4 cup fresh berries of your choice.

Instructions:

Place the yogurt in a bowl or glass. Top with the granola and fresh berries. Serve.

Prep time: 5 minutes

9. Turkey Apple Wrap:

Ingredients:

1 whole wheat wrap

2 ounces cooked deli turkey

1/4 cup diced apple

1/4 cup shredded lettuce

1 tablespoon mayonnaise

1 tablespoon honey mustard.

Instructions:

Place the wrap on a plate. Top with the turkey, apple, lettuce, mayonnaise and honey mustard. Roll up the wrap and cut in half. Serve. **Prep time**: 5 minutes

10. Hummus and Veggie Pita:

Ingredients:

1 whole wheat pita

2 tablespoons hummus

1/4 cup diced vegetables of your choice (e.g., carrots, peppers, cucumber).

Instructions:

Spread the hummus on the pita. Top with the diced vegetables. Cut the pita in half and serve. **Prep time**: 5 minutes

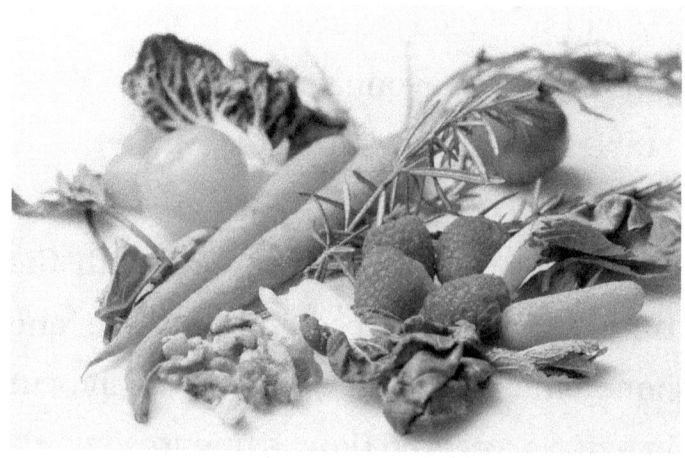

CHAPTER 10

Healthy Pregnancy Recipes

Dinner

1. Baked Salmon with Sweet Potatoes and Green Beans

Ingredients:

- 2 salmon filets
- 2 sweet potatoes, cut into cubes
- 2 cups green beans
- 2 tablespoons olive oil
- 2 tablespoons honey
- 2 tablespoons of oregano
- 1 teaspoon of garlic powder
- Salt and pepper to taste

Instructions:

- Preheat the oven to 375 F.

• Place the salmon filets on a baking sheet lined with parchment paper.

• In a large bowl, combine the sweet potatoes, green beans, olive oil, honey, oregano, garlic powder, salt, and pepper.

• Mix everything together until all the vegetables are evenly coated.

• Place the vegetables around the salmon and bake for 15-20 minutes, or until the vegetables are tender and the salmon is cooked through.

• Serve and enjoy!

Prep Time: 10 minutes

Cook Time: 20 minutes

2. Spinach and Ricotta Stuffed Shells

Ingredients :

• 1 box of jumbo shell pasta

• 2 tablespoons olive oil

- 1 onion, diced
- 2 cloves garlic, minced
- 4 cups spinach
- 1 container of ricotta cheese
- 2 cups marinara sauce
- 1 cup shredded mozzarella cheese

Instructions:

- Preheat the oven to 375 F.
- Bring a pot of salted water to a boil and add the shells. Cook for 8-10 minutes until al dente. Drain and set aside.
- Heat the olive oil in a skillet over medium heat. Add the onion and garlic and cook until softened.
- Add the spinach and cook until wilted.
- In a large bowl, mix together the ricotta cheese, spinach mixture, and 1/2 cup of the marinara sauce.
- Stuff each shell with the ricotta mixture and place them in a 9×13 inch baking dish.

· Top the shells with the remaining marinara sauce and mozzarella cheese.

· Bake for 25 minutes.

· Serve and enjoy!

Prep Time: 15 minutes

Cook Time: 35 minutes

3. Quinoa, Black Bean, and Corn Salad

Ingredients:

· 1 cup quinoa

· 2 cups vegetable broth

· 1 can black beans, rinsed and drained

· 1 cup corn

· 1 red bell pepper, diced

· 1 jalapeno, minced

· 2 tablespoons olive oil

· Juice of 1 lime

· 2 tablespoons honey

· 2 tablespoons cilantro

· Salt and pepper to taste

Instruction:

· Bring the vegetable broth to a boil in a medium saucepan.

· Add the quinoa and reduce heat to a simmer. Cook for 15 minutes or until the quinoa is cooked through.

· In a large bowl, combine the cooked quinoa, black beans, corn, bell pepper, and jalapeno.

· In a small bowl, whisk together the olive oil, lime juice, honey, cilantro, salt, and pepper.

· Pour the dressing over the quinoa mixture and toss to combine.

· Serve and enjoy!

Prep Time: 10 minutes

Cook Time: 15 minutes

4. Roasted Vegetable and Hummus Wrap

Ingredients:

· 4 whole wheat tortillas

· 1 can chickpeas, drained and rinsed

· 1 red bell pepper, cut into cubes

· 1 zucchini, cut into cubes

· 1 yellow squash, cut into cubes

· 2 tablespoons olive oil

· 1/2 teaspoon garlic powder

· 1/2 teaspoon oregano

· Salt and pepper to taste

· 1/2 cup hummus

Instructions:

· Preheat the oven to 375 F.

· Place the bell pepper, zucchini, and squash on a baking sheet lined with parchment paper.

· Drizzle with olive oil and season with garlic powder, oregano, salt, and pepper.

- Roast for 20-25 minutes, or until the vegetables are tender.
- In a food processor, combine the chickpeas, garlic powder, oregano, salt, and pepper and process until smooth.
- Spread the hummus on each tortilla and top with the roasted vegetables.
- Roll up the tortillas and enjoy!

Prep Time: 10 minutes

Cook Time: 25 minutes

5. Baked Zucchini Fritters

Ingredients

- 2 zucchinis, grated
- 2 eggs
- 1/4 cup all-purpose flour
- 1/4 cup grated Parmesan cheese
- 1/2 teaspoon garlic powder
- 1/2 teaspoon onion powder
- Salt and pepper to taste

· 2 tablespoons olive oil

Instructions:

· Preheat the oven to 375 F.

· Place the grated zucchini in a strainer and sprinkle with salt. Let sit for 10 minutes.

· Squeeze out the excess moisture from the zucchini and place in a bowl.

· Add the eggs, flour, Parmesan cheese, garlic powder, onion powder, salt, and pepper and mix until combined.

· Heat the olive oil in a skillet over medium heat.

· Drop spoonfuls of the zucchini mixture into the skillet and cook for about 3 minutes per side, or until golden brown.

· Transfer the fritters to a baking sheet lined with parchment paper.

· Bake for 15 minutes, or until cooked through.

· Serve and enjoy!

Prep Time: 10 minutes

Cook Time: 25 minutes

6. Baked Sweet Potato Fries

Ingredients:

- 4 sweet potatoes, cut into fries
- 2 tablespoons olive oil
- 1 teaspoon garlic powder
- 1 teaspoon paprika
- Salt and pepper to taste

Instructions:

- Preheat the oven to 375 F.
- Place the sweet potato fries on a baking sheet lined with parchment paper.
- Drizzle with olive oil and season with garlic powder, paprika, salt, and pepper.
- Bake for 20-25 minutes, or until golden brown and crispy.
- Serve and enjoy!

Prep Time: 10 minutes

Cook Time: 25 minutes

7. Vegetable Fried Rice

Ingredients:

· 2 tablespoons olive oil

· 1 onion, diced

· 2 cloves garlic, minced

· 2 cups cooked brown rice

· 1 cup frozen vegetables

· 2 eggs

· 2 tablespoons soy sauce

Instructions:

· Heat the olive oil in a large skillet over medium heat.

· Add the onion and garlic and cook until softened.

· Add the cooked rice and frozen vegetables and cook for 3-4 minutes.

- Push the rice mixture to one side of the skillet and crack the eggs into the other side.
- Cook the eggs until scrambled, then mix everything together.
- Add the soy sauce and cook for an additional 2 minutes.
- Serve and enjoy!

Prep Time: 10 minutes

Cook Time: 15 minutes

8. Baked Teriyaki Chicken

Ingredients:
- 2 boneless, skinless chicken breasts
- 1/2 cup teriyaki sauce
- 2 tablespoons olive oil
- 2 cloves garlic, minced
- 1 teaspoon ginger, minced
- Salt and pepper to taste

Instructions:

· Preheat the oven to 375 F.

· Place the chicken breasts in a baking dish.

· In a small bowl, whisk together the teriyaki sauce, olive oil, garlic, ginger, salt, and pepper.

· Pour the teriyaki mixture over the chicken breasts and bake for 25-30 minutes, or until the chicken is cooked through.

· Serve and enjoy!

Prep Time: 10 minutes

Cook Time: 30 minutes

9. Eggplant Parmesan

Ingredients:

· 1 eggplant, sliced into rounds

· 2 tablespoons olive oil

· 2 cups marinara sauce

- 1 cup shredded mozzarella cheese
- 1/2 cup grated Parmesan cheese
- Salt and pepper to taste

Instructions:

- Preheat the oven to 375 F.
- Place the eggplant rounds on a baking sheet lined with parchment paper.
- Drizzle with olive oil and season with salt and pepper.
- Bake for 15 minutes, or until golden brown.
- Spread 1/2 cup of the marinara sauce on the bottom of a 9×13 inch baking dish.
- Place the eggplant rounds on top of the marinara sauce.
- Top with the remaining marinara sauce and sprinkle with the mozzarella and Parmesan cheese.
- Bake for 15 minutes, or until the cheese is melted and bubbly.
- Serve and enjoy!

Prep Time: 10 minutes

Cook Time: 30 minutes

10. Lentil Soup

Ingredients:

· 2 tablespoons olive oil

· 1 onion, diced

· 2 cloves garlic, minced

· 2 carrots, diced

· 2 stalks celery, diced

· 1 teaspoon oregano

· 2 cups dry lentils

· 6 cups vegetable broth

· Salt and pepper to taste

Instructions:

· Heat the olive oil in a large pot over medium heat.

· Add the onion, garlic, carrots, and celery and cook until softened.

• Add the oregano and lentils and cook for 1 minute.

• Add the vegetable broth and bring to a boil.

• Reduce heat to a simmer and cook for 25-30 minutes, or until the lentils are cooked through.

• Season with salt and pepper.

• Serve and enjoy!

Prep Time: 10 minutes

Cook Time: 35 minutes

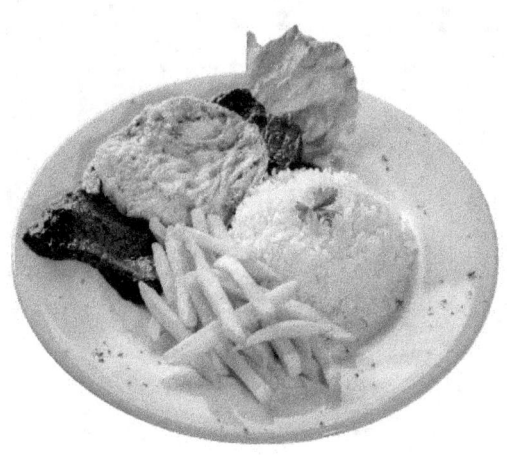

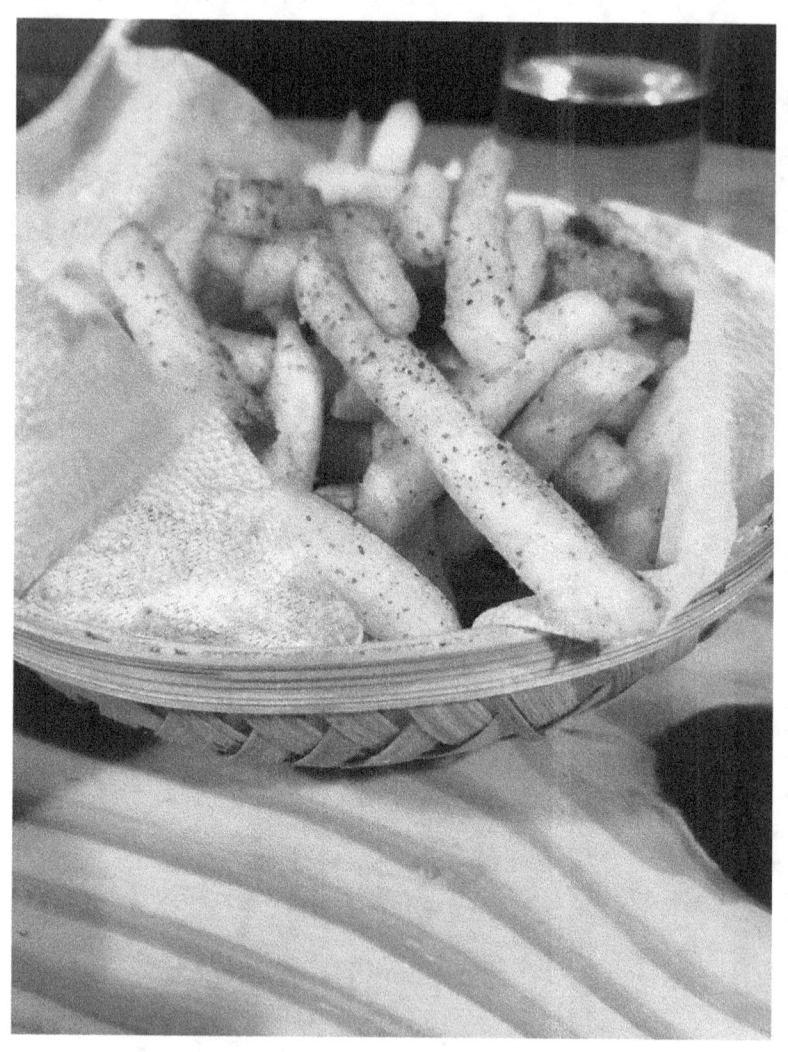

CHAPTER 11

Healthy Pregnancy Recipes

Snacks

1.Greek Yogurt Parfait

Ingredients:

1 cup Greek yogurt

1/2 cup mixed berries

2 tablespoons honey

2 tablespoons chopped almonds

Instructions:

1. In a bowl, combine Greek yogurt, berries, honey, and almonds.

2. Mix well until the ingredients are evenly distributed.

3. Serve and enjoy!

Prep Time:5 minutes

2. Crunchy Apple Slaw

Ingredients:

1 apple, cored and sliced

1/4 cup shredded carrots

1/4 cup shredded cabbage

2 tablespoons olive oil

1 tablespoon lemon juice

1/2 teaspoon honey

1/4 teaspoon ground cinnamon

Instructions:

1. In a large bowl, combine apple, carrots, and cabbage.

2. In a small bowl, whisk together olive oil, lemon juice, honey, and cinnamon.

3. Pour over the apple mixture and toss to coat.

4. Serve and enjoy!

Prep Time: 10 minutes

3. Avocado Toast

Ingredients:

2 slices whole-grain bread

1/2 avocado, mashed

1/4 teaspoon garlic powder

1/4 teaspoon smoked paprika

Instructions:

1. Toast the bread until golden and crisp.

2. Spread mashed avocado over the toast.

3. Sprinkle garlic powder and smoked paprika over the avocado.

4. Serve and enjoy!

Prep Time: 5 minutes

4. Roasted Chickpeas

Ingredients:

1 can chickpeas, drained and rinsed

1 tablespoon olive oil

1/2 teaspoon garlic powder

1/2 teaspoon paprika

1/2 teaspoon ground cumin

Instructions:

1. Preheat the oven to 375°F.

2. Spread the chickpeas on a baking sheet and drizzle with olive oil.

3. Sprinkle it with garlic powder, paprika, and cumin.

4. Roast for 15 minutes, stirring once or twice.

5. Let cool before serving.

 Prep Time: 15 minutes

5. Trail Mix

Ingredients:

1/4 cup roasted almonds

1/4 cup roasted cashews

1/4 cup dried cranberries

1/4 cup raisins

Instructions:

1. In a bowl, combine almonds, cashews, cranberries, and raisins.

2. Mix until evenly distributed.

3. Serve and enjoy!

Prep Time:5 minute

6. Sweet Potato Fries

Ingredients:

1 large sweet potato, cut into fries

1 tablespoon olive oil

1/4 teaspoon garlic powder

1/4 teaspoon smoked paprika

Instructions:

1. Preheat the oven to 375°F.

2. Spread the sweet potato fries on a baking sheet and drizzle with olive oil.

3. Sprinkle it with garlic powder and smoked paprika.

4. Bake for 25 minutes, flipping once halfway through.

5. Serve and enjoy!

Prep Time: 25 minutes

7. Mediterranean Veggie Wrap

Ingredients:

1 whole-wheat wrap

1/4 cup hummus

1/4 cup diced tomatoes

1/4 cup diced cucumbers

1/4 cup crumbled feta cheese

Instructions:

1. Spread the wrap with hummus.

2. Top with tomatoes, cucumbers, and feta cheese.

3. Roll up and enjoy!

Prep Time: 10 minutes

8. Baked Zucchini Chips

Ingredients:

1 large zucchini, sliced

1 tablespoon olive oil

1/4 teaspoon garlic powder

1/4 teaspoon dried oregano

Instructions:

1. Preheat the oven to 375°F.

2. Spread the zucchini slices on a baking sheet and drizzle with olive oil.

3. Sprinkle it with garlic powder and oregano.

4. Bake for 20 minutes, flipping once halfway through.

5. Serve and enjoy!

Prep Time: 20 minutes

9. Veggie Hummus Plate

Ingredients:

1/4 cup hummus

1 cup sliced bell peppers

1 cup sliced cucumbers

1/4 cup crumbled feta cheese

Instructions:

1. Spread the hummus on a plate.

2. Arrange the bell peppers, cucumbers, and feta cheese around the hummus.

3. Serve and enjoy!

Prep Time: 10 minutes

10. Banana-Chocolate Chip Muffins

Ingredients:

2 ripe bananas, mashed

1/4 cup melted butter

1/2 cup sugar

1 teaspoon vanilla extract

1 egg

1 cup all-purpose flour

1 teaspoon baking powder

1/4 teaspoon baking soda

1/2 cup semi-sweet chocolate chips

Instructions:

1. Preheat the oven to 350°F.

2. In a large bowl, combine mashed bananas, melted butter, sugar, vanilla extract, and egg.

3. In a separate bowl, whisk together flour, baking powder, and baking soda.

4. Add the flour mixture to the banana mixture and stir until just combined.

5. Fold in the chocolate chips.

6. Divide the batter into a 12-cup muffin tin and bake for 25 minutes.

7.let cool before serving

PrepTime:25 minute

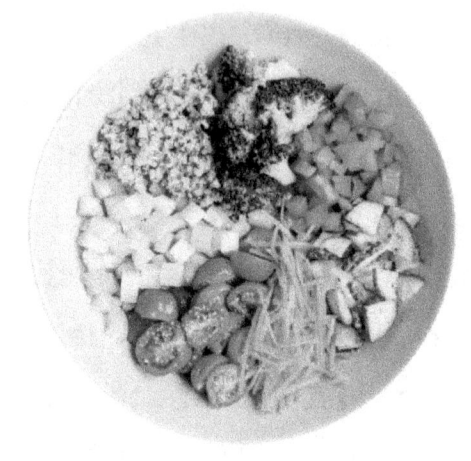

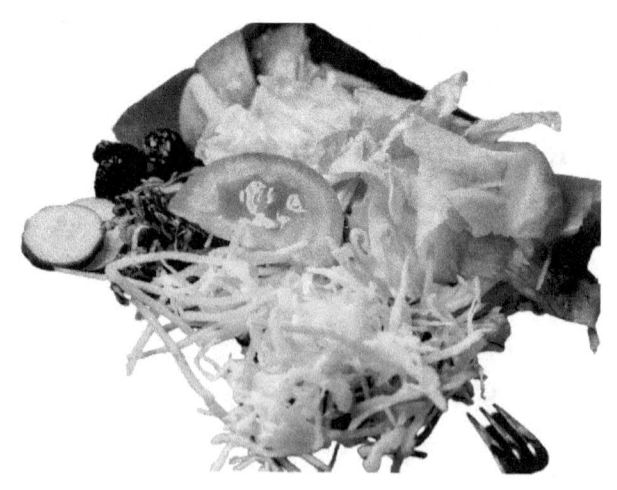

90

CONCLUSION

This pregnancy diet cookbook is an invaluable resource for any expecting mother looking to maintain a healthy and balanced diet during pregnancy. It provides an array of delicious and nutritious recipes that are easy to make and can help keep the mother and baby healthy throughout the pregnancy. It also offers helpful advice on what to eat, when to eat, and how to adjust the food choices to meet the mother's individual needs. With this book, pregnant women can make well-informed decisions about their diet and ensure that they are getting all the nutrients they need to have a healthy and happy pregnancy.

This Pregnancy Diet Cookbook is an essential resource for pregnant women looking to eat healthy and nutritious meals during their pregnancy. With over 100 recipes to choose from, this book provides an array of delicious and nutritious meals that are easy to make and provide the essential vitamins and minerals needed for a healthy pregnancy. The book includes recipes for breakfast, lunch, dinner, snacks, and desserts, as well as helpful tips for eating out, shopping for groceries, and meal planning.

The recipes in this cookbook are tailored for pregnant women, who need additional vitamins and minerals to support the development of their baby. All the recipes are easy to make, with few ingredients and simple instructions. Many of the recipes use nutritious ingredients such as lean proteins, fresh fruits and vegetables, whole grains, and dairy. This book is a great resource for pregnant women looking to make sure they are getting the nutrition they need during pregnancy.

By following the recipes in this book, pregnant women can ensure they are getting the nutrition they need to have a healthy pregnancy and a healthy baby.

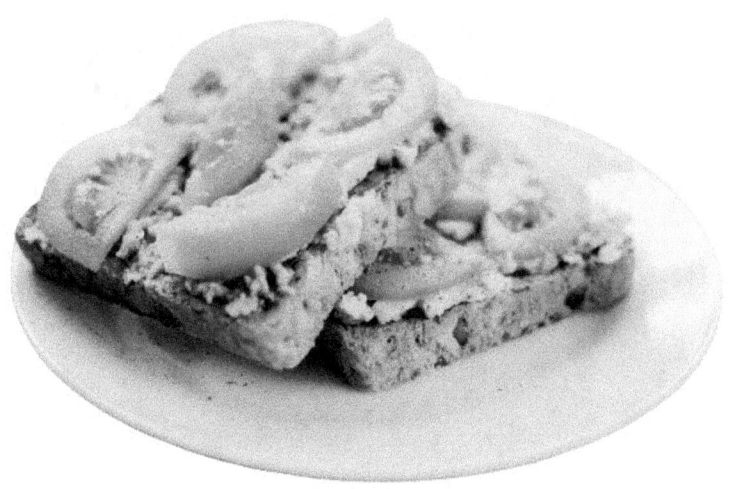

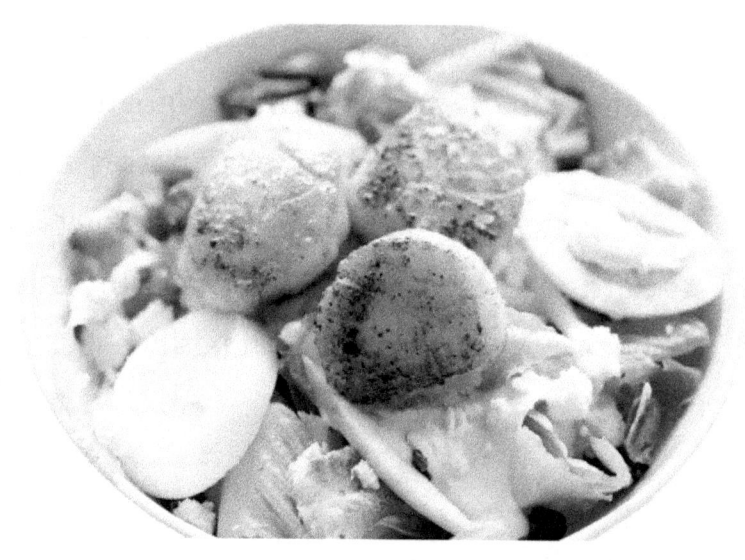

www.ingramcontent.com/pod-product-compliance
Lightning Source LLC
Chambersburg PA
CBHW070748220526
45467CB00018B/1455